Gastric Sleeve Surgery in Mexico

HOW I LOST
179 POUNDS

BRANDI CARTER

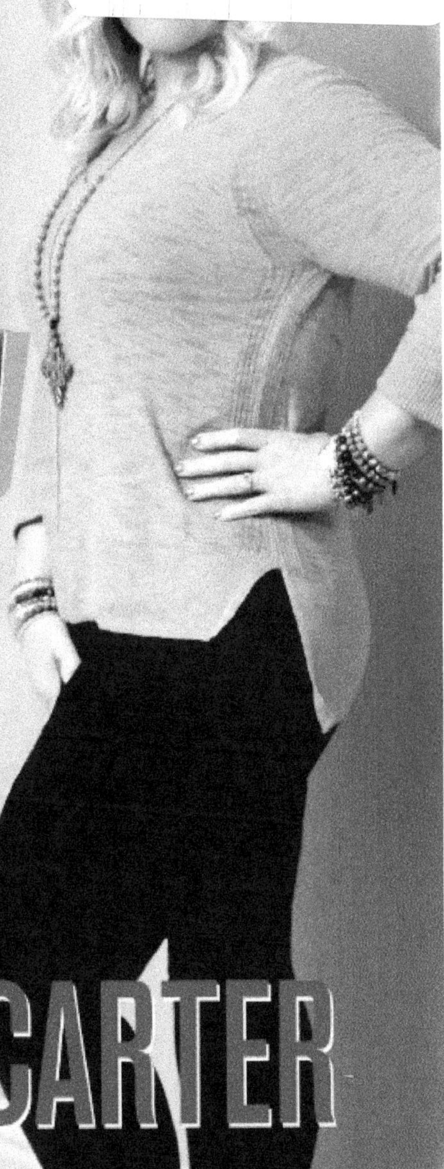

Copyright © 2018 by Brandi Carter

All rights Reserved

No part of this book may be used or reproduced in any manner whatsoever without written permission of the author.

Printed in the United States of America

ISBN: 978-1717214300

Easy Read Publishers
4000 E. Bristol Street, Suite 3
Elkhart, IN 46514

Table of Contents

Dedication

I would like to dedicate this book to the memory of my beautiful mother who was my best friend; the memory of my amazing Gammie, my grandmother, who was also my best friend, and who always tried to teach me to do what was right; my awesome sisters for taking this VSG journey with me; my wonderful husband and two sons who will always love and support me;

And last but not least, to Dr. A for saving my life. I am forever grateful for the life that you and your surgical skill have given back to me.

Chapter 1

Addicted to food

People who have never had an addiction don't understand how hard it can be.

Payne Stewart

Why is food so addictive? Is there something in food that just comforts our soul? I'm not quite sure on the answer to that, but I do know one thing...

I am a food addict!

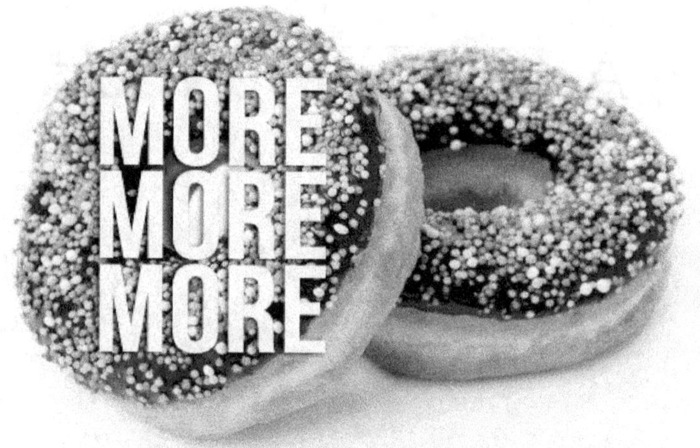

There are many forms of addiction. Most of them can be stopped abruptly and although you will have side effects, you can still live. With food addiction, you can't just stop eating. It's something our body needs for survival. This makes it much harder to control this terrible addiction.

No matter where I am or what I'm doing; my addiction will always follow me.

For as long as I can remember I have always been overweight. Food has always been a big part of our family life causing the entire family to be overweight.

- Eat to celebrate.
- Eat to drown out pain.
- Eat when you feel happy.
- Eat when life is throwing you curves
- Eat – just because.

My parents divorced when I was young, my sister Holly and I would spend a lot of weekends at my grandparents' home.

My Gammie was my everything.

She was a huge Weight Watchers fan. She tried to teach me about diet and exercise. She counted and weighed just about everything. After eating we'd go for a long walk; sometimes twice a day. I loved being with my grandparents. But I always looked forward to going home again so I could eat anything and everything I wanted.

I remember on the weekends my papa would often cook us pancakes with lots of butter and the edges would be crisp, or white rice with butter, milk, and sugar.

Gammie would let us eat what papa cooked for us but we knew we'd go for a walk afterwards.

They lived in a very small farm town, and we would walk the block, and then walk around the cemetery. That might sound crazy, but it was like a beautiful park. I learned to love those walks – even as an 8-year-old.

Dessert at Gammie's

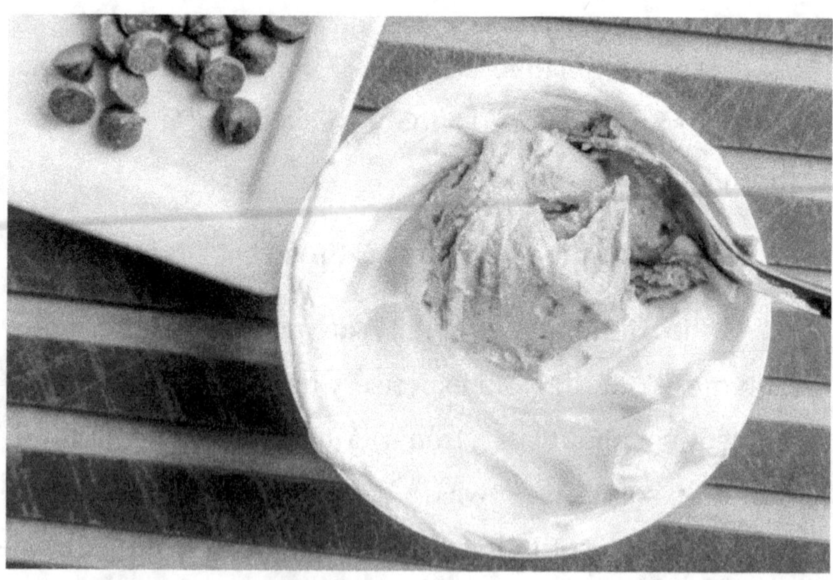

For dessert at her house, we would have 2 big tablespoons of frozen yogurt with 1 tablespoon of peanut butter. She measured everything. She was very adamant about feeding us healthy and making sure we didn't overeat.

She tried to teach us healthy eating habits, but the draw to food was too strong.

It didn't help that as soon as I got home, there was anything and everything to eat. It didn't matter who's house I was at – my entire family loved food.

I lived most of the time with my mother and step-father. Mom was big with hamburger helper, chicken fried steak, minute steaks with gravy, and the always easy-to-get Kentucky Fried Chicken. She often worked two jobs, so she tried doing the quickest option.

My step mom was a great cook also. Any time we would go to dad's house, there was always a 4-course southern style meal.

For holidays, I didn't have just one place to go, I had three places to go.

Food was a big thing and I learned to binge eat going from home to home. I took a plate home with me from each house, which was over filled because I would say it is for my entire family. Sometimes I would even hide food so I could eat it at a later time. I remember sneaking food in my backpack or my purse as I got in Jr. High.

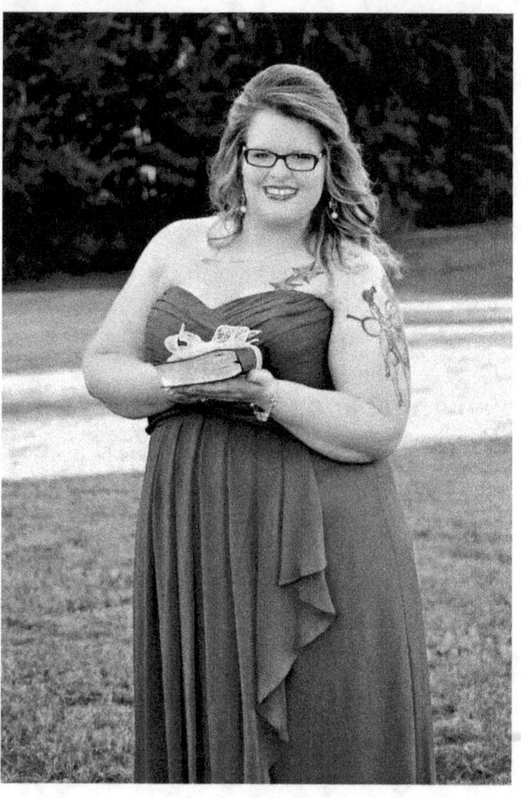

Months after my VSG I was down 50+ lbs and found my mother's Bible. Here I am at my beautiful sister's wedding. I was proud to carry it as she was my "reason" for having my surgery and saving my life.

It was a habit I kept up through the years. Even after I was married, I would go to the grocery store, buy a big king-size candy bars and hide them in my purse. Any time my husband or my son wasn't around, I would eat them.

I was ashamed of what I was doing, and I knew better. Now, I'm not saying a person can't have a candy bar every now and then. But, I was eating a meal along with desert then still eating a candy bar afterwards. There is something wrong with that picture and I knew it.

As I got older, the hide and eat secret got worse and worse.

Chapter 2

Family History

Like most overweight people, I had to hit rock bottom before I'd take responsibility for the consequences of neglecting my own health '.

-- Stephen Furst

B oth of my parent were morbidly obese. My father, aka Big Poppa, is a big man at 6' 3" and 350 + pounds. He has had 2 heart attacks, and also type 2-diabetes. My mother always weighed around 320 and was 5'5". I'm not sure of her exact weight at death, but at 56 years old, a massive heart attack took her life.

She never had signs of heart issues, but at her weight, I now know it was simply a matter of time.

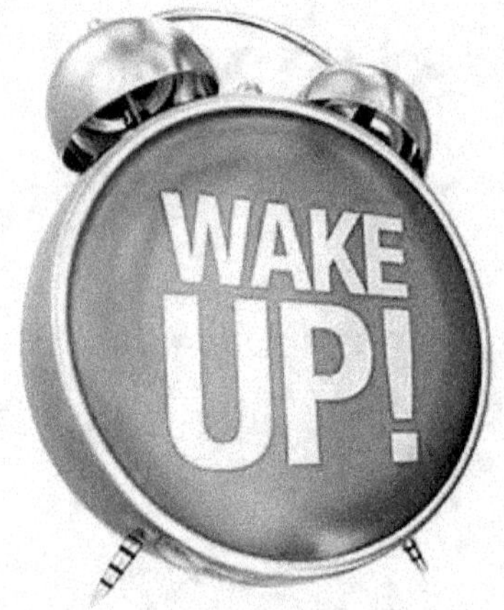

My wakeup call: It was my mom's obesity that killed her, and I was headed down the same road

At my first obstetrician visit, at 19 years old, I weighed 220 pounds. Throughout the pregnancy, I had gained an immense amount of weight.

In only 9 short months, when I went into the hospital to give birth to my first son, Christian, I weighed 306.

After I had him, I only lost 15 pounds.

I tried getting back on track with Weight Watchers, along with my grandma. I just never seemed to be able to stay focused and committed to it.

I tell people all the time - food is a drug. It's no different than a crackhead needing their crack. A food addict needs their food, and it was a drug for me.

I tried everything.

I also went to the doctor, he put me on Phentermine pills.

I loved the way the Phentermine made me feel.

Since I was eating three and four thousand calories a day I didn't have much energy.

The Phentermine gave me energy I needed.

I did manage to lose about 60 pounds while being on the pills.

But soon after the weight would creep back up because the pills no longer worked like they did in the beginning.

Chapter 3

Could it work for me?

I never worry about diets. The only carrots that interest me are the number you get in a diamond.

-- Mae West

You name the diet and I've tried it. I'd lose some and then gain that and more back.

When I had my second son, Aiden, I started out at 325 pounds but only gained 18 pounds with him.

I ended up joining a local Fitness Bootcamp program shortly after Aiden was born.

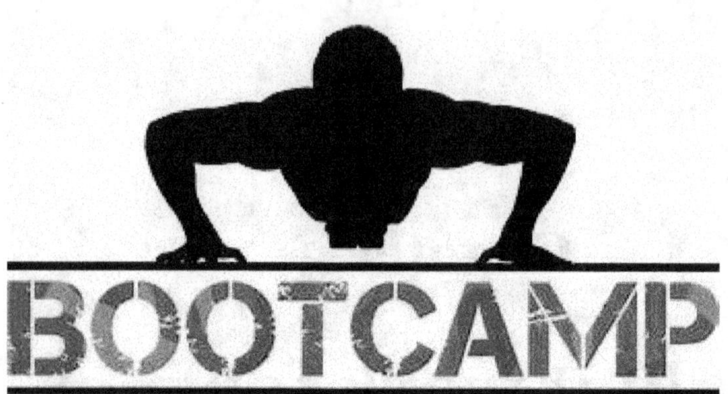

I Lost 65 Pounds

The owners talked with me about my weight and helped me realize that I did have a issue and needed to get it fixed.

The owner confronted me in a way no one ever had. He put it in perspective to me. "Do you want to leave your kids here at a young age? Because you're going to die."

I didn't know this man from Adam at this time, but he came to me and said it to me in a way that slapped me in the face and woke me up.

This was in 2014.

When he said that to me, it did a lot for me.

It made me grow in a different way than anybody who has approached me with weight loss.

Through their training and exercise I lost over 65 pounds and I was much leaner than I've ever been.

I loved every minute of it, but I was still morbidly obese

The pain my body endured during work outs soon caught up to me.

The scale was not moving fast enough and I gave up.

I ballooned back up to 400 pounds quickly

I joined a local clinic run by a physician who was well known for helping people lose a lot of weight.

He told me I was pre diabetic and my best bet was to do his liquid diet program.

He started me on a 600-calorie liquid diet along with a diet pill.

He told me from the beginning, some people just need bariatric surgery to help get them past the point of where they always stop.

Some people need the tool to assist them in their journey.

You could potentially be one of those people.

Over the next couple years I did research on bariatric surgery. I quickly ruled out a Gastric Bypass or the Lapland.

There were too many complications for me to consider either of these two options.

It was then I found the surgery I felt was right for me: Gastric Sleeve. More formally called, the Vertical Gastric Sleeve Surgery.

Dr. Alvarez in Mexico

I was a hairdresser at the time, which connected me with a lot of people and their stories.

One of my clients had weight loss surgery and I watched her go from a size 24 to a size 5.

She transformed right before my eyes.

I wanted that same transformation so I began to do more research on weight loss surgery.

She had surgery performed by a local surgeon who no longer did surgery here. I looked into the other local doctor, which did not have the best reviews because of multiple reasons. As I continued my journey in search for the perfect surgeon for me I met a sweet lady name Brooksie on Facebook.

She had nothing but praises about Dr. Guillermo Alvarez – a surgeon from Mexico.

Soon after I met a beautiful soul name Tessa in the salon I work at.

She sang nothing but praises on Dr. Alvarez and staff with their medical skills.

It was then I began my search in earnest.

Never would I have thought of having surgery in Mexico, but I kept seeing one name come up over and over: Dr. Guillermo Alvarez in Mexico. The same doctor who Brooksie and Tessa had mentioned.

It was about that time my mother died of the heart attack. I knew something had to change. I had tried diets, gyms, boot camps, and online workouts. They'd work for a while and then I'd pack the weight right back plus more.

I began to ask questions of other people who'd had weight loss surgery and again Dr. Alvarez's name kept coming up over and over again.

It was time to search more about this doctor.

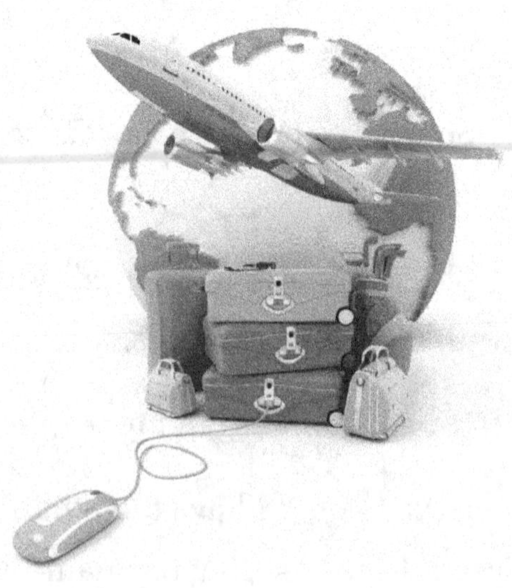

Chapter 4

Mexico? You've got to be kidding

Judgment is judgment, whether you're obese, or too skinny, or not athletic enough.

-- Anna Kournikova

I had never thought about going to Mexico for surgery.

Even at 418 pounds, I did not have any apparent health issues so my insurance would not approve surgery.

I knew that I would be paying for the surgery myself no matter which surgeon I chose.

It took me a little time to get over the feeling of failure. Failure that I could not lose weight "the normal way."

But the more I spoke with other people who'd had surgery (most with Dr. Alvarez) the more I realized diet and exercise just doesn't work for some people – and I was one of them.

Since then I've found out that Dr. Alvarez has performed weight loss surgery on over 1,500 people from our area alone!

Suddenly, going to Mexico sounded like a real possibility.

Once you find one of Dr. Alvarez's patients, it will lead you to as many others as you care to talk to (he's performed over 12,500 surgeries).

I also learned that THE only surgery he performs is the Gastric Sleeve surgery.

No lap band.

No gastric bypass.

His reasoning: it's the safest and easiest for the patient with long term great results. And there is not the issue with malnutrition like with the gastric bypass.

That made sense to me because that is what I had decided from my own research.

I began to call patients

I wasn't satisfied with what I read online. Or the conversations I'd had with Brooksie and Tessa. I had to talk to as many patients as I could to find out "the real story."

So I began to make calls.

I talked to people all over the world over the next month or two.

I estimated I spoke with 100 people or more who had had surgery with Dr. Alvarez.

But besides speaking with patients who'd already had surgery, I began to search the internet – looking for the bad things people were saying about Dr. Alvarez.

I know that sounds terrible, but I wanted to hear something bad. I wanted to KNOW- what could be the worst that could happen to me if I went to Mexico for surgery?

I found nothing.

Not one person had made bad remarks about Dr. Alvarez anywhere. I stayed up countless nights searching... all to find nothing but good things said about him.

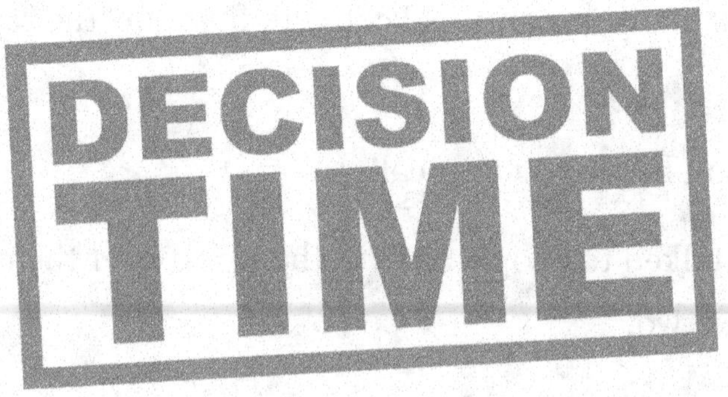

Before I made my final decision, I had to be sure my primary physician was on board, so I made an appointment for my yearly physical.

He had also been my mother's primary doctor. Just like the man from fitness boot camp was straight up with me, my primary doctor is the same way. He tells me how it is. He doesn't sugar-coat anything.

He said to me "*you're going to end up just like your mom if you do not do something about it.*"

"*I've told you this over the past two years, and I'm going to tell you again, I send a lot of my patients to Dr. Alvarez in Mexico, and every one of them has turned out great. So, you really need to consider it.*"

I confessed that I had already talked to over 100 people over the last year or so. I've looked for things that are bad and I couldn't find them."

He said "*You're not going to. That's who he is. That's why I'm telling you that you need to go and see him for that reason.*"

I said something to him about the money situation and he said "*how do you eat a hippo?*"

I looked at him like he was crazy.

He said "*one day at a time.*" He said "*that's what you're going to do with that payment, one day at a time.*"

I had been thinking negatively, but he confirmed that he would take care of me if something happened. Of course, that fully sealed the deal for me.

I left there with the confidence of knowing he's got my back 100%. (*I learned from some Facebook groups not all primary physicians are as supportive of their patients having surgery in Mexico. But then, those doctors don't know Dr. Alvarez*).

I applied for and got my financing approved for surgery- next step, scheduling my surgery.

My sister decided to join me on the surgical journey and scheduled her surgery for the same day. Her husband decided to go along with us, so the three of us packed our car to make the 14 hour drive to Eagle Pass, Texas – where Dr. Alvarez's transportation driver, Rosy, picked us up to take us on the 1 mile trip across the border to the hospital.

(NOTE TO FUTURE PATIENTS: that was a crazy decision. 14 hours is a long enough drive with 3 people in

the car but coming back right after surgery was not fun. Don't do it.)

People, all the time, are bragging and talking big about going on vacations in Mexico, and how beautiful and how "I would love to go back and stay longer" and yet when I talk about going to Mexico for weight loss surgery they kind of freak out. Why? If they can take their family to Mexico, what's so different to go there for a medical procedure?

Now, I agree – not all places give world class care or have world class technique as Dr. Alvarez. But neither do all the surgeons and hospitals in the US.

You need to do your homework like I did

Chapter 5

Not all Surgeons from Mexico Are As Skilled

If you walk down the street, within five minutes you will see someone who is morbidly obese or obese.

-- Carnie Wilson

I paid $8,900 for my surgery. You can get the Gastric Sleeve surgery done for around $4,000 in other places in Mexico.

But Google those places. You'll find out

- you are there for 1 day and then sent away on your own

- Or your surgery is done in a strip mall

- Or you are just a number – one of 13 surgeries to be performed that day

- Or that surgeon has had serious complications

I was NOT looking for a Walmart price or a Walmart cheap experience.

I wanted THE best and was willing to pay more for it in Mexico, but far, far less than if I had had it done in the US.

Ask yourself these questions about the $4,000 Mexican places

- What are they NOT doing to make it cheaper?

- What older technique/technology are they using to cut corners?

- Is a junior surgeon performing the surgery with less experience?

- Will they answer your questions after you leave?

- What is their complication rate?

- Will they support you if there are complications?

- How much information do they provide to their patients?

- Can you speak to your surgeon when you get home?

- Will you have his/her phone number and email and if so, will they respond in a timely manner?

- How many patients have lost their lives using these other surgeons?

- How do they pay their staff with $4,000-5,000 and still give you an effective surgery?

You get what you pay for is certainly true for surgery in Mexico.

I wasn't willing to take play the risk game for surgery in Mexico just to save a few dollars. This is my life we are talking about! And my future!!

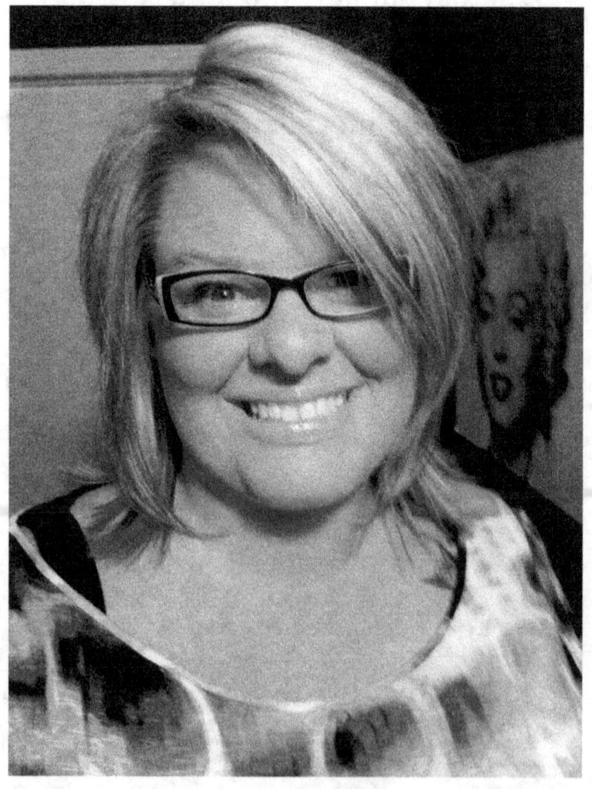

Trying to smile through the pain of my own problem - my weight.

Chapter 6

I Finally Meet Dr. Alvarez

The interesting thing about overeating or being obese is there's this physical manifestation of it.

-- Jami Attenberg

When we met Dr. A (that's what all his patients call him) I was expecting someone that's not real fluent in English. Even though I had watched several of his YouTube videos before I went, I still didn't know what to expect.

I was astonished.

His English was flawless (I found out later he went to school through Junior High in Eagle Pass, Texas so speaks and writes English like a native).

When I talked with him, it was just like talking to one of my friends.

There was no uneasy feeling.

I knew instantly I had made the right decision coming to Mexico and having surgery with Dr. A.

I had a notebook paper full of questions for him. You would have thought I'd have all the questions answered by that time. I'd spoken to over 100 people and Susan – his patient coordinator – many times.

But that's just who I am.

But Dr. A grabbed his cup of coffee had a seat and smiled at me and said let's hear them.

He answered all of my questions without making me feel I was wasting his time.

It so different from what I experienced in my hometown with the surgeon at the meeting there.

Dr. Alvarez just built a 5-star hospital/medical center. Since it wasn't built yet, we had surgery in a local privately-owned hospital. It's not as modern as the hospital in my hometown, but the nurses were great and very attentive.

Of course, the surgical team with Dr. Alvarez leading them is world class as well.

After we were weighed and our pictures taken we walked to the lab area where our blood was drawn and chest x-rays taken.

Once we were done in the lab, it was off to our hospital room.

They were sweet enough to put my sister and I in a double room.

I was the last one to go for surgery that day so it gave me time to put my phone on the charger, lay out my nightgown, and arrange my pillow and blanket (I know, I know – I didn't need to bring a blanket and pillow but since we drove I did it to make me more comfortable).

When I came out of surgery, I looked at my brother-in-law and sister and said "when are they going to take me?"

He said "You've already had surgery." I said "no, they haven't taken me back yet." He said "yes, they have."

I had to raise my gown up and check my stomach to see for myself that surgery had already been done. I didn't feel any pain and couldn't remember a thing.

I got up shortly after to go to the restroom and the left side of my stomach felt as if I had done a whole lot of crunches. Some people may call it pain, but I felt that it was just uncomfortable.

I never had nausea.

I had a little bit of a gas but it didn't last long.

Dr. Alvarez had told my sister and I to get up and walk as soon as we felt alert enough to. That it would help to remove the excess gas from surgery. I walked those halls every 30 minutes until I went to bed that night.

I know everyone's experience is different, but I can tell you after having talked with 150 people or so that this is normal for Dr. A's patients, but not so normal with other surgeons. You're monitored carefully the whole time you're there and checked frequently by Dr. A and his assisting surgeons/doctors. I never once felt uncomfortable, afraid, or nervous.

**All I could think about was that I was on the loser's bench.
My new life had begun!**

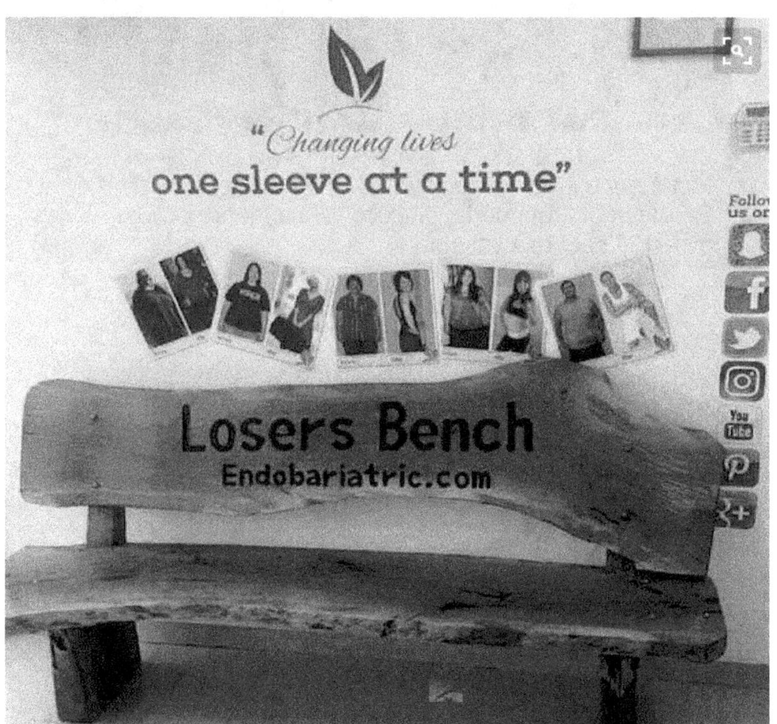

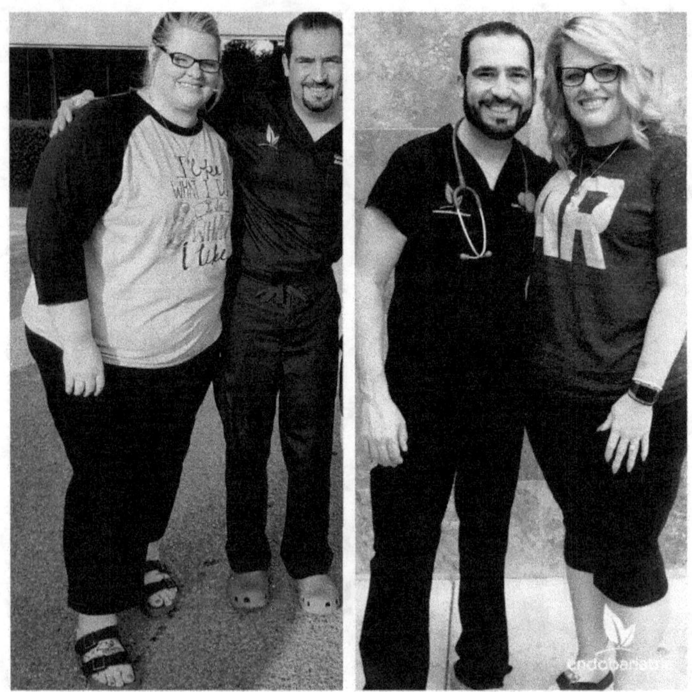

Picture of the left is the day I left Mexico after surgery.
On the right I returned to Mexico with a friend. Down
over 150 pounds by then.

Chapter 7

Life After Surgery

Very often, overweight children have parents who are struggling with weight issues.

-- Lisa Ling

At 400 pounds I had to do 30 days of a pre-opt diet to shrink my liver so there'd be room to work on my stomach. That was the hardest part of the whole thing for a food addict like me.

But, once surgery was over, I had no problem following Dr. A's guidelines to the T.

In the hospital on day 2, I was given some ice chips that I had to just let melt. The cold water would go into my swollen stomach and begin the healing process.

Of course, I was on a 3-day regimen of antibiotics and sent home with pain medicine and anti-acids with strict instructions to take all the anti-acids.

On day 2 my sister, brother-in-law and I went in the Endobariatric van for a trip to the city market. I felt fine. It was a great experience.

Who would have thought I'd be out shopping 1 day after surgery. It was an awesome experience to see all the local things and experience their culture.

As I walked around shopping, I thought: Could I really lose weight or would I be one of the ones this surgery would not work for?

On day 3 we were released for the long 14-hour drive back home.

I've never seen a doctor give so much information to his patients as Dr. A. We had a printed document that told us what to eat over the next 4 weeks.

We also got a reminder email at the end of each week when it was time to begin the next eating phase.

And if that's not enough, there is a very active – and supportive – private Facebook group that encourages and answers non-medical related questions. Any medical questions are answered via email by Dr. A or Susan.

Dr. A even shoots a weekly #AskDr.A show when he answers any and every question we might have.

11,500+ had traveled this journey ahead of me as patients with Dr. A. I figured if they could succeed, I could too.

And succeed I have.

179 pounds and still going.

What so great about a smaller stomach is that you fill up fast. It's like having the bumpers up on a bowling alley. You can never get a gutter ball. But it doesn't mean you'll get a strike.

With the sleeve I'll never be able to stuff myself. But it doesn't mean I can't make bad choices. I still have to use the tool and choose wisely.

But I am so thankful for this tool.

I continue to be amazed. I was a very sick person before. My immune system was low. Being a cosmetologist, I was around every illness out there.

I used to have strep throat about four or five times a year, sinus infections at least every three months, bronchitis, double pneumonia, and ear infections in both ears.

Since surgery I may have been sick twice and neither one of them were antibiotics sick. One time, I had a little fluid in my ear that was bothering me, and the other time, my allergies were acting up. It's been amazing.

My primary physician was right about the $220 per month I had to pay for the loan for my surgery. I've had no problem making the payment because

- I've saved money from doctor visits
- I've saved (big time) money on food

Many people reduce or eliminate their medications and save money there too.

It's affected my whole family. My oldest son was obese also and we were making plans to have him go for surgery. But since I've been home and changed my meals, my family has eaten differently also.

- My son has lost 70 pounds (without surgery).
- My husband has lost 50 pounds (no surgery either)

Our whole family is healthier and more active than ever before

A lot of people do not understand that when I say this I don't mean that it's an easy surgery.

It's a simple surgery for us, as the patient. You're not cut open from hip to hip and from rib bone to hip bone. People think that all the time.

When they talk about my surgery, "I can't believe you went back to work after five days." I'm like "listen, it was a simple surgery, I'm just tired."

I've even shown my stomach. It was not a pretty by any means. There were five little bitty scars and that's it.

Another question people ask me is if I feel like just another paycheck for Dr. Alvarez.

My answer is a resounding NO!

I probably would have if I had gone ahead with the local surgeon, but certainly not with Dr. A.

He only does three people or the occasional fourth one each day – which gives him time to give us personal attention.

Even after surgery, we stayed in contact. I could still, to this day, any time I wanted to, message him, or e-mail him, which, I know he prefers. He's very, very involved with his patients and he wants his patients to be successful. It's not just about the paycheck for him.

Of course, everybody must get a paycheck, but this is his heart. This is his soul.

If you're successful, he's successful and that's the way he sees it in his eyes.

I know that, I could tell that from the time I met him. I told him all the time, he's my hero, and I don't think he gets it. He's that to so many people. I don't think that he understands how much people look up to him and appreciate what he does for all of us.

He doesn't just do it for us. He does it for our kids, he does it for our husbands and wives, and the rest of the people that we're around.

I'm a better person for my friends, family, and coworkers, I can help them more, because I'm have more energy in me since losing the weight. If can help make the next person be more successful, that is what my heart desired, because that is what he did that for me.

Since Day 1 I have posted on social media about my journey. I have been an open book for so many people. My inbox and text messaging blew up constantly with messages and questions. I have and will always help anyone that needs assistance in this journey. It has been such a blessing to me that if I could help the next person win the battle against obesity that is what I wanted to do.

I had video interviews with Dr. A's team, phone interviews; I was even interviewed by ABC news at one point.

For almost a year I did this day in and day out. I sent so many people to Dr. A. for their VSG surgery. I was asked on several occasions, "Do you get paid to do this?" My answer: "No, I do this because my heart knows the pain of obesity. I know what Endobariatric, Dr. Alvarez, and Susan has done for my life. I just want to reach out a helping hand to the Endobariatric team and save more lives if I could at all costs.

It wasn't long, Dr. Alvarez noticed my social media pages were steady with questions and answers about him and his team. I always answered people back with my truth. I never "sugar coat" anything. He let me know what I was doing did not go unnoticed and he appreciated what I was doing to help others fight obesity.

May 2016, I had a conversation with Dr. Alvarez and little did I know my entire life was about to change for the better. I was offered a position in being part of the best bariatric team in the entire world!

I was now Endobariatrics patient assistant!

I also help with managing social media groups.

I have never felt so honored and blessed in my entire life.

Now on to helping save even more lives because now I have the key to success being a part of Dr. A and his flawless team.

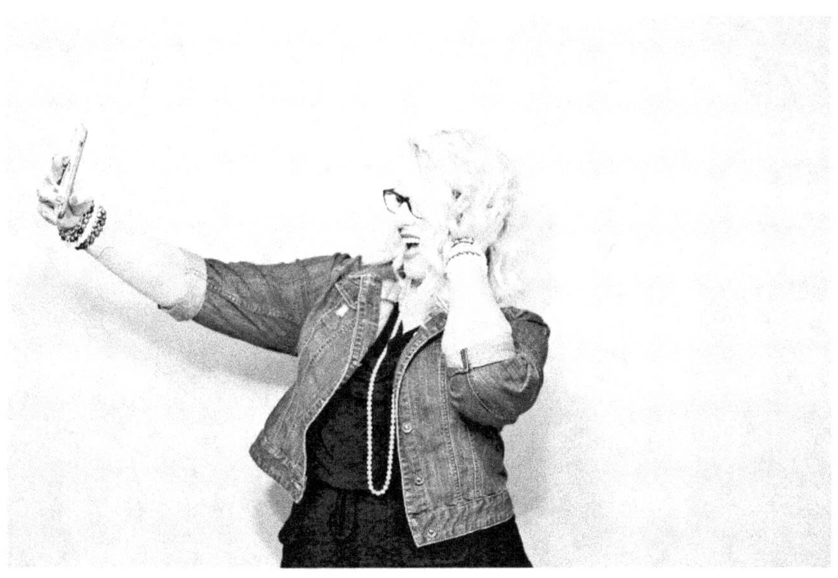

Life is good when you like what you see in the mirror.

Chapter 8

My Journey Back To Mexico

When you reduce your body mass you will start to notice you're feeling more energetic. That's those hormones kicking in – getting you back on track.

-- Dr. Guillermo Alvarez

Fourteen months after my sister Holly and I had surgery, our younger sister, Raeann, decided to have VSG surgery as well. After her search, looking for her perfect surgeon she decided to go through her insurance and go locally. I went with her to all of her appointments at the local surgeon's clinic including a bariatric seminar he held. I had a notebook full of questions and as soon as I got to question #2 he told me I'd have to just come in for a private office visit. Of course one I would have to pay for.

I don't think he liked me asking questions in a public arrangement.

He was pushing the bypass surgery, and you could tell he didn't have confidence in talking about the gastric sleeve. Not that he couldn't do it, but just that he doesn't recommend it, and he couldn't give a logical reason why he couldn't recommend it.

- When I asked him about the size of the stomach, which was my very first question I asked him, of course he said it was a 36 bougie that he used (the form used when crafting a gastric sleeve). I knew Dr. Alvarez uses a 32 – which is smaller.

- Second question: "how come you choose to use the bigger ones? Why would you want your patients to have a bigger stomach?"

To me that meant not as successful in the long run.

In my mind I was thinking, "Why would you just take a little bit out? Why wouldn't you take more to help your patients be more successful?"

I guess that was none of my business and he needed me/my sister, to make an appointment to answer that question because he didn't answer it for me.

I knew right then and there I did not want my baby sister to use the local surgeon at all. She on the other hand, did not know as much about the surgery and decided to pursue it further.

She was told her insurance would cover all but $1200-1800 by his patient coordinator days later on the telephone. She went ahead and scheduled the appointment to get it all set up. He sent her to a physiatrist, which cost her money for a psych evaluation. Also, to her primary doctor for a release and letter stating she needed the surgery for medical reasons.

Again, being supportive I went with her.

Little did I know we would be face to face with the man who did not like me questioning him about his surgical skill.

At this point he had no idea I had already had surgery. I was about 165 lbs. down from 418 lbs., so I was still over weight.

He was asking her questions and I stayed quiet.

My momma and gammie taught me if I had nothing nice to say, then say nothing at all.

He kept directing things to her about her support system. I felt he should1 have just asked- "who are you and would you be supportive of what she is doing?" She told him I was her big sister, that I have had VSG surgery already and have been extremely successful.

Curious George came out in him and he needed to know where I had surgery, and with who. I respectfully said "not here".

He kind of laughed and said but where? My sister spoke up and said "in Mexico".

He laughed and said yea I have fixed many of those cases.

Well he had lit a fire in me after that. First, I just cannot believe the bedside manner of some doctors to down grade another doctor and at this point he had no idea who did my surgery. In the short time I have worked with Dr. A learning Endobariatric and the inside detail, I have never heard him be in the slightest disrespectful to another bariatric surgeon.

But don't worry I sure let him know a thing or two, respectfully.

"You may have fixed many of those, but none from my surgeon, Dr. Guillermo Alvarez. He is a world-renowned surgeon. Dr. Alvarez is one of 11 surgeons in the world that hold the title of Master Surgeon in Metabolic and Bariatric Surgery.

He does not have those type of problems you are referring to sir.

You can see his record it is public. He has done well over 12,500+ surgeries."

The room got silent for a second. My sister looked at me like I KNOW YOU DIDN'T JUST SAY ALL THAT TO THIS MAN... But she knows me well enough; if you step on my toes I will let you know about it. Therefore I had to let him know.

He moved forward with the visit and sent us to schedule her surgery.

I didn't know it then, but I now know that was the best gift he could have ever given my sister because it made things clearer for her to use Dr. Alvarez. His clinic let her know as we left that day

- she would have to sign an 18-month contract to visit his office 12 times at $35 each.
- She would have to purchase her pre-opt liquid diet food from his office at $300.
- Attend any nutrition classes if he felt necessary/post-opt.
- Plus, a $5000 deposit to the hospital. She may get some of that back and may not.

As soon as we step outside she was in tears because her feelings of not being able to have the surgery she felt was over. Sissy saved the day because I was on the phone with the amazing Susan George (Dr. A's patient coordinator) and we were scheduling her surgery with Dr. Alvarez.

She went to her local bank got financing and she was set to go!

I went along with her. And I got to experience what very few people get to experience: I got to be in the operating room to watch and Snap Chat her entire surgery!

It was a mind boggling to watch the magic take place.

I get a lot of questions

I get a lot of questions about the actual surgery. Now I was going to watch my sister's surgery first hand and I would have so many more answers for Dr. A's patients. I was thrilled.

I remember going to sleep when I had my tonsils taken out at age 30. There was so much chaos and just clanking of things and it just being uncomfortable.

I wondered what all the noise was about.

There was none of that with Dr. A.

It was so smooth.

Everyone knew what to do, where to be, what he needed and when.

There were several nurses, 2 surgeons (besides Dr. A), 1 general doctor to assist, and 1 anesthesiologist. Most of them have been with Dr. A through all those 12,500+ surgeries.

The years of surgical experience in that operating room was astonishing.

After the patient has been prepped, the lights dim, and he listens to music while he's forming the sleeve.

Focused.

Precise.

Confident.

No distractions.

Happy he's changing another life.

I smiled as he moved his feet and legs a little bit. Not really dancing, but you could just feel the confidence in himself and knowing the happiness and the joy he's getting from saving her life.

30 minutes later surgery was over.

Everybody says he runs like a well-oiled machine and you have no idea until you've sat and watched him do that.

We have good surgeons here in the US, but I'm so thankful for that first Facebook message to Brooksie because I didn't just get a good surgeon, I got THE BEST.

I owe my life and the life of my family to one amazing, caring, talented bariatric surgeon in Mexico: Dr. Guillermo Alvarez, a third generation surgeon.

Thank you from the bottom of my heart!

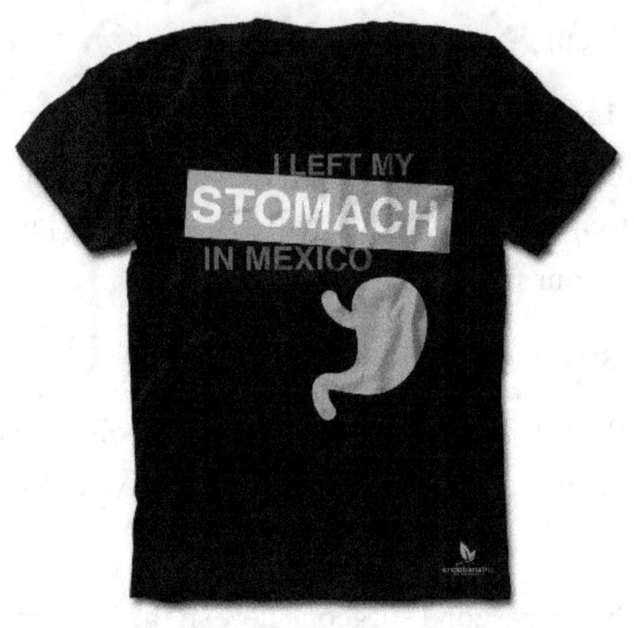
I LEFT MY
STOMACH
IN MEXICO

65

Chapter 9

Epilog

Now that I've lost 179 pounds (and still losing) life is much different. I have much more stamina and I can do things I never could do before.

I've quit trying to find anything negative about this surgery (and of course Dr. Alvarez) and enjoying my new much thinner life.

I know it's possible that if you're reading this book or listening to the CD with it, that you are in the same position I was. You may not be 400 pounds, but you're overweight, obese or maybe even morbidly obese.

You feel awful.

You want to hide from cameras.

You're tired of yo-yo dieting.

Your health may be deteriorating.

You're embarrassed.

Your joints hurt.

You can't do things with your children or grandchildren like you wish you could.

Hopefully my story, my journey will be an inspiration for you. That it will encourage you to check out the gastric sleeve surgery as a possible option.

And to check out having it with Dr. Alvarez.

I am 100% convinced there is no better surgeon for this surgery on the planet. When that's all he does 3-4 times a day 5 times a week for years, he has fine-tuned it to near perfection.

And when you care as much as he does about all his patients, there is no price tag that can be put on that.

If there's anything I can do. Any question I can answer, I'd be happy to chat with you.

Email me at Brandi@Endobariatric.com

I'm here for you.
Brandi Carter,
Jonesboro, Arkansas

418 pounds and miserable!

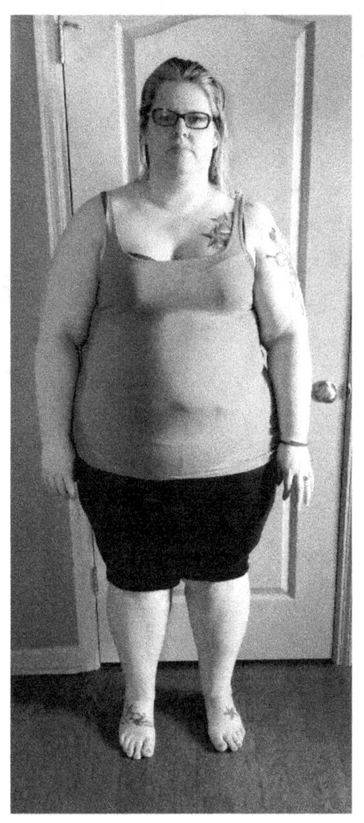 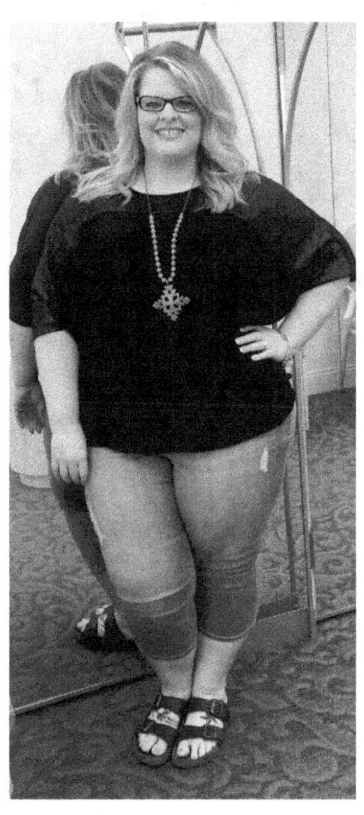

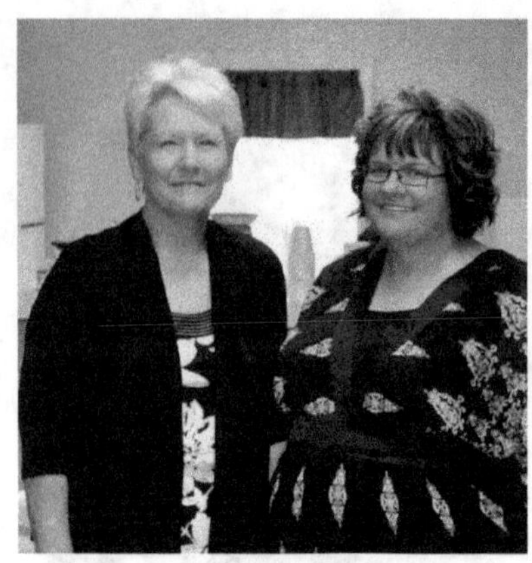
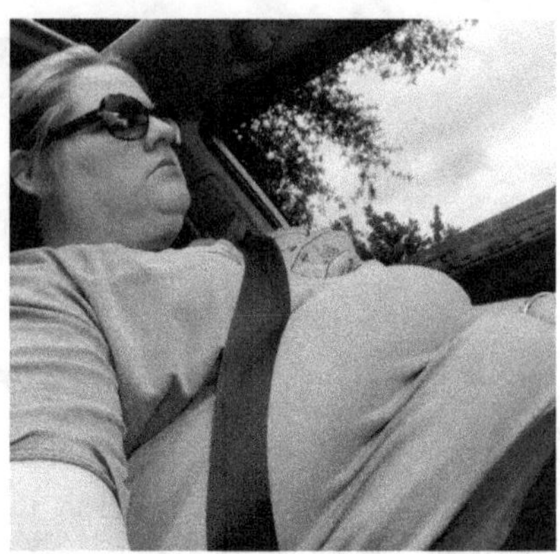

At 5' 11" and 239 pounds!

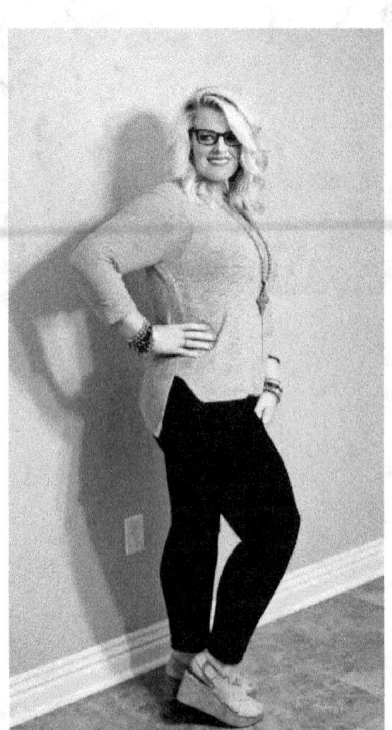